Keto Diet Recipes

Easy Keto Diet Cookbook with 50 Wholesome Low-Carb Recipes you'll want to Make Everyday

Ketogenic Lifestyle

Healthy Keto Food pyramid

Berries

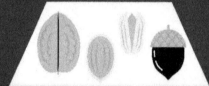
Nuts and seeds

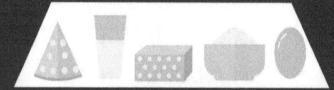
Full Fat Dairy and eggs

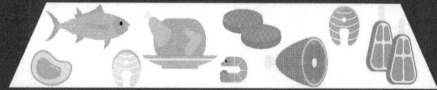
Meat and fish

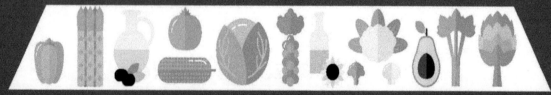
Vegetables low in carbs and oils

© Copyright 2021 by Ketogenic Lifestyle - All rights reserved.

The following Book is reproduced below with the goal of providing information that is as accurate and reliable as possible. Regardless, purchasing this Book can be seen as consent to the fact that both the publisher and the author of this book are in no way experts on the topics discussed within and that any recommendations or suggestions that are made herein are for entertainment purposes only. Professionals should be consulted as needed prior to undertaking any of the action endorsed herein.

This declaration is deemed fair and valid by both the American Bar Association and the Committee of Publishers Association and is legally binding throughout the United States.

Furthermore, the transmission, duplication, or reproduction of any of the following work including specific information will be considered an illegal act irrespective of if it is done electronically or in print. This extends to creating a secondary or tertiary copy of the work or a recorded copy and is only allowed with the express written consent from the Publisher. All additional right reserved.

The information in the following pages is broadly considered a truthful and accurate account of facts and as such, any inattention, use, or misuse of the information in question by the reader will render any resulting actions solely under their purview. There are no scenarios in which the publisher or the original author of this work can be in any fashion deemed liable for any hardship or damages that may befall them after undertaking information described herein.

Additionally, the information in the following pages is intended only for informational purposes and should thus be thought of as universal. As befitting its nature, it is presented without assurance regarding its prolonged validity or interim quality. Trademarks that are mentioned are done without written consent and can in no way be considered an endorsement from the trademark holder.

Table of Contents

Introduction..10

Chapter 1. Breakfast 13
1. Keto Cheese Chips 14
2. Kale, Edamame and Tofu Curry 15
3. Bacon Appetizers...17
4. Antipasti Skewers 18
5. Rosemary Lamb Chops 20
6. Grilled Pork Spare Ribs..21
7. Pork and Beef Meatballs 22
8. Hearty Pork Stew Meat...23

Chapter 2. Mains 25
9. Turkey Chili 26
10. Keto Wraps with Cream Cheese and Salmon.....................28
11. Tuna Casserole 30
12. Keto Red Curry 31

Chapter 3. Sides...33
13. Creamy Kale Salad 34
14. Brussels sprouts with Bacon 36
15. Bacon Mashed Cauliflower 37
16. Grilled Mediterranean Veggies 39
17. BLT Salad Preparation..41
18. Crab Cakes with Almond Flour 43

Chapter 4. Seafood..44
19. Quick Butter Cod 45
20. Creamy Mackerel 46
21. Herb Crusted Tilapia 47
22. Shrimp Avocado Salad 48

Chapter 5. Poultry..49
23. Parmesan Chicken 50
24. Chili Lime Chicken with Coleslaw.......................................52

25. Lemongrass Chicken 53
26. Crispy Crust Whole Chicken 55

Chapter 6. Meat 57
27. Greek-Style Cold Beef Salad 58
28. Beef Wellington 60
29. Oven Roasted Rib-Eye Steak 62
30. Stuffed Tomatoes with Cotija Cheese 63
31. Coconut Fajita Chicken 65

Chapter 7. Vegetables 66
32. Low-carb cheesy omelet 67
33. Margherita Mushroom Pizza 69
34. Cauliflower, leeks and broccoli 71
35. Braised Fennel with Lemon 73
36. Easy Summer Vegetable Medley 75

Chapter 8. Soups and Stews 77
37. Bacon Green Soup 78
38. Zucchini and Celery Soup 80
39. Turkey Taco Soup 81
40. Tomato Soup 82
41. Cheesy Cauliflower Soup 83
42. Hot Mushroom Clear Soup 84

Chapter 9. Snacks 85
43. Country Style Chard 86
44. Bacon-Wrapped Sausage Skewers 87
45. Apple Crisp 88
46. Sugar Snap Bacon 90

Chapter 10. Desserts 91
47. Chocolate Peanut Butter Ice Cream Bars 92
48. Crockpot Apple Pudding Cake 94
49. Mocha Ice Bombs 96
50. Dark Chocolate Almond Bark 97

Conclusion 100

Introduction

The keto diet is the latest diet craze, and it's certainly a great one. The keto diet was first developed in the 1950s by Dr. Robert Atkins to treat his own epilepsy, but today, just about anything can be classified as a "keto" diet.

The ketogenic diet works by drastically reducing carbohydrates in the diet. When this occurs, the liver converts fat into ketone bodies, which are used for energy by every cell in your body. The body then makes use of these ketones, often referred to as "ketones" and "ketone bodies," through a process called "beta-oxidation" to produce energy (ATP) that's not reliant on insulin.

You can lose weight and enjoy the benefits of a keto diet without having to have a radical change in lifestyle. Ketosis is a natural physiological state that your body enters when in ketosis. When your body is in ketosis, it begins burning fat for energy rather than using sugar.

That's great news for your health, but what if you don't like eating meat or other animal products? You don't have to worry! While many people think of low-carb diets as being low in protein, people on a keto diet actually consume more protein than they typically would on a standard American diet.

When you eliminate carbs from your diet, some people will find that they are able to drop some weight quickly.

Most carb-free diets will not be as effective as a low-carb diet when it comes to losing weight, but for those who wish to eliminate carbs for other reasons, adopting a keto diet could be the answer to their problems.A keto diet restricts carbohydrates to the point where the body eventually begins to break down and burn fat as fuel. The result is weight loss and better overall health. This book covers everything related to the ketogenic diet, including what it is, what it does.As you can imagine, this is a state where the body uses fat as its primary source of energy instead of sugar or carbohydrates. Although the name may sound intimidating, it's actually quite simple to follow. You will begin by restricting carbohydrates to less than 50 grams per day, which is about six to nine teaspoons for most people. It's been used to treat epilepsy, cancer, and many other health conditions. To learn more about the benefits of the ketogenic meal plan, read on to learn more about the ketogenic diet. When you are committed to a KETO DIET, you want to make it as easy as possible to follow the diet. That is why we made the Keto Diet Cookbook.You can use the Keto Diet Cookbook for daily meals or as a reference guide during your diet. The Keto Diet Cookbook includes recipes that are easily prepared with ingredients you probably already have around the house.

Chapter 1. Breakfast

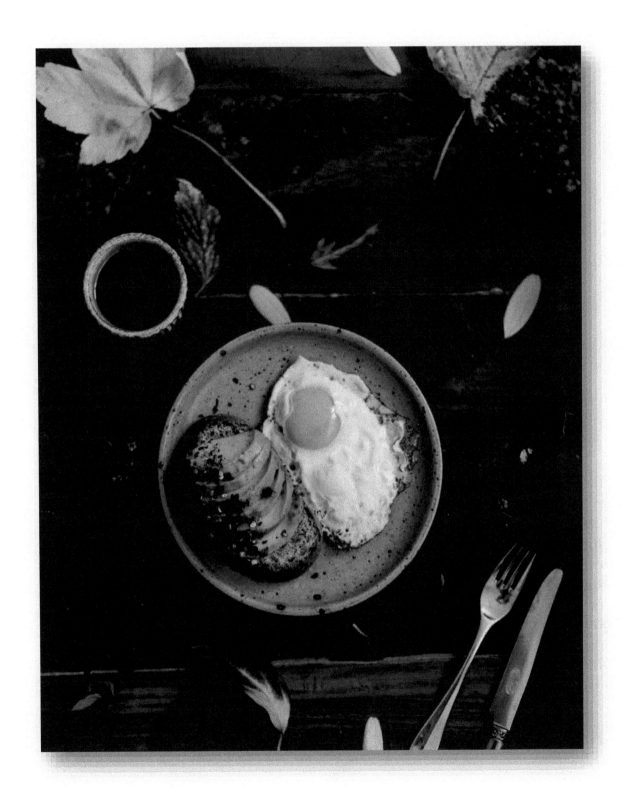

1. Keto Cheese Chips

Preparation Time: 10 minutes

Cooking Time: 10 minutes

Servings: 3

Ingredients:

- 1 ½ cups cheddar cheese, shredded
- 3 tablespoons ground flaxseed meal
- Garlic salt to taste

Directions:

1. Preheat your oven to 425 degrees F.
2. Create a small pile of 2 tablespoons cheddar cheese on a baking sheet.
3. Sprinkle flaxseed on top of each chip.
4. Season with garlic salt.
5. Bake in the oven for 10 minutes.
6. Let cool before serving. Nutrition:

Calories 288 Total Fat 22.2g

Saturated Fat 11.9g Cholesterol 59mg Sodium 356mg

Total Carbohydrate 5.8g Dietary Fiber 4g

Total Sugars 0.3g Protein 17.1g Potassium 57mg

2. Kale, Edamame and Tofu Curry

Preparation Time: 20 minutes

Cooking time: 40 minutes

Servings: 3

Ingredients:

- 1 tablespoon rapeseed oil
- 1 large onion, chopped
- Four cloves garlic, peeled and grated
- 1 large thumb (7cm) fresh ginger, peeled and grated
- 1 red chili, deseeded and thinly sliced
- 1/2 teaspoon ground turmeric
- 1/4 teaspoon cayenne pepper
- 1 teaspoon paprika
- 1/2 teaspoon ground cumin
- 1 teaspoon salt
- 250 g / 9 oz. dried red lentils
- 1-liter boiling water
- 50 g / 1.7 oz. frozen soya beans
- 200 g / 7 oz. firm tofu, chopped into cubes
- Two tomatoes, roughly chopped
- Juice of 1 lime
- 200 g / 7 oz. kale leaves stalk removed and torn

Directions:

1. Put the oil in a pan over low heat. Add your onion and cook for 5 minutes before adding the garlic, ginger, and chili and cooking for a further 2 minutes. Add your turmeric, cayenne, paprika, cumin, and salt and Stir through before adding the red lentils and stir it again.

2. Pour in the boiling water and allow it to simmer for 10 minutes, reduce the heat and cook for about 20-30 minutes until the curry has a thick '•porridge' consistency.

3. Add your tomatoes, tofu and soya beans and cook for a further 5 minutes. Add your kale leaves and lime juice and cook until the kale is just tender. Nutrition:

Calories 133

Carbohydrate 54

Protein 43

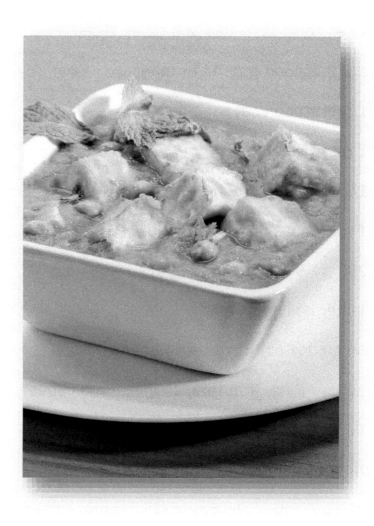

3. Bacon Appetizers

Preparation Time: 15 minutes

Cooking Time: 2 hours

Servings: 6

Ingredients:

- 1 pack Keto crackers
- ¾ cup Parmesan cheese, grated
- 1 lb. bacon, sliced thinly

Directions:

1. Preheat your oven to 250 degrees F.
2. Arrange the crackers on a baking sheet.
3. Sprinkle cheese on top of each cracker.
4. Wrap each cracker with the bacon.
5. Bake in the oven for 2 hours.

Nutrition:

Calories 440 Total Fat 33.4g Saturated Fat 11g Cholesterol 86mg

Sodium 1813mg

Total Carbohydrate 3.7g Dietary Fiber 0.1g

Total Sugars 0.1g Protein 29.4g Potassium 432mg

4. Antipasti Skewers

Preparation Time: 10 minutes

Servings: 6

Ingredients:

- 6 small mozzarella balls
- 1 tablespoon olive oil
- Salt to taste
- 1/8 teaspoon dried oregano
- 2 roasted yellow peppers, sliced into strips and rolled
- 6 cherry tomatoes
- 6 green olives, pitted
- 6 Kalamata olives pitted
- 2 artichoke hearts, sliced into wedges
- 6 slices salami, rolled
- 6 leaves fresh basil Directions:

1. Toss the mozzarella balls in olive oil.
2. Season with salt and oregano.
3. Thread the mozzarella balls and the rest of the ingredients onto skewers.
4. Serve on a platter. Nutrition:

Calories 180 Total Fat 11.8g

Saturated Fat 4.5g Cholesterol 26mg Sodium 482mg

Total Carbohydrate 11.7g

Dietary Fiber 4.8g Total Sugars 4.1g Protein 9.2g Potassium 538mg

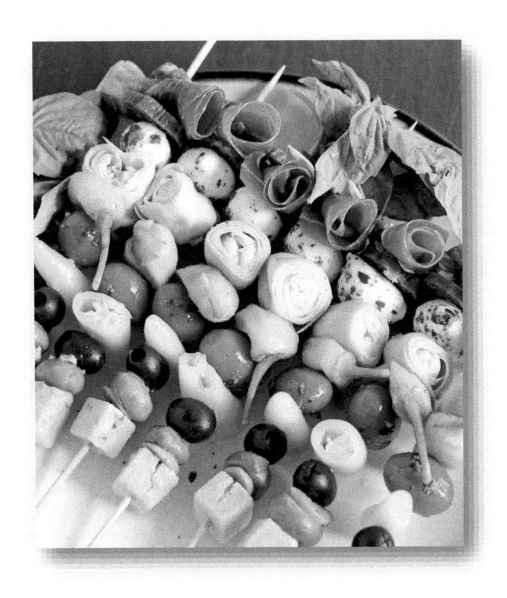

5. Rosemary Lamb Chops

Preparation time: 1 hour

Cooking Time: 2 hr.

Servings: 3 Ingredients:

- 3 crushed garlic cloves
- 1 t. salt
- 1 tbsp. of each:
- Cayenne pepper
- Freshly crushed rosemary
- Freshly crushed thyme leaves
- ½ c. olive oil
- 3 (1 ½-inch) lamb loin chops Directions:

1. Combine the spices (rosemary, thyme, cayenne, and salt) with the garlic and oil. Mix well and add the chops. Coat the pork thoroughly and let it marinate in the fridge for 1 hour.

2. After that time, add the fixings to a large Sous Vide bag and seal.

3. Submerge in the prepared cooker (154ºF) for 2 hours.

4. Open the bag and serve with your favorite side dishes.

Nutrition:

Calories: 242 Fat: 13 g Net Carbs: 0 g

Protein: 29.4 g

6. Grilled Pork Spare Ribs

Preparation time: 10 minutes

Cooking time: 50 minutes

Servings: 4

Ingredients:

- 1 tablespoon erythritol
- Salt and black pepper, to taste
- 1 tablespoon olive oil
- 1 teaspoon chipotle powder
- 1 teaspoon garlic powder
- 1-pound (454 g) pork spare ribs
- 1 tablespoon sugar-free BBQ sauce

+ extra for serving Directions:

1. Mix the erythritol, salt, pepper, oil, chipotle, and garlic powder. Brush on the meaty sides of the ribs, and wrap in foil. Sit for 30 minutes to marinate.

2. Preheat oven to 400ºF (205ºC), place wrapped ribs on a baking sheet, and cook for 40 minutes to be cooked through. Remove ribs and aluminum foil, brush with BBQ sauce, and brown under the broiler for 10 minutes on both sides. Slice and serve with extra BBQ sauce and lettuce tomato salad.

Nutrition:

Calories: 294 fat: 18g protein: 28g carbs: 3g net carbs: 3g fiber: 0g

7. Pork and Beef Meatballs

Preparation time: 5 minutes

Cooking time: 13 minutes

Servings: 5

Ingredients:

- 1-pound (454 g) ground pork
- ½ pound (227 g) ground beef
- Onion, chopped
- Garlic cloves, minced
- 1 teaspoon Hungarian spice blend Directions:

1. In a mixing bowl, thoroughly combine all ingredients until they are well incorporated. Form the mixture into meatballs with oiled hands. Place your meatballs on a tinfoil-lined baking sheet.

2. Bake in the preheated oven at 395ºF (202ºC) for 12 to 14 minutes or until they are golden brown.

3. Arrange on a nice serving platter and serve. Bon appétit!

Nutrition:

Calories: 377 fat: 24g protein: 36g carbs: 2g net carbs: 2g fiber: go

8. Hearty Pork Stew Meat

Preparation time: 10 minutes

Cooking time: 1 hour

Servings: 5 Ingredients:

- 2 tablespoons olive oil
- 2 pounds pork stew meat
- 1 yellow onion, chopped
- 1 garlic clove, minced
- ¼ cup dry sherry wine
- 4 cups chicken bone broth
- 1 cup tomatoes, pureed
- 1 bay laurel
- Sea salt and ground black pepper, to taste
- 1 tablespoon fresh cilantro, chopped

Directions:

1. Heat the olive oil in a soup pot over a moderate flame. Sear the pork for about 5 minutes, stirring continuously to ensure even cooking; reserve.

2. Cook the yellow onion in the pan drippings until just tender and translucent. Stir in the garlic and continue to sauté for a further 30 seconds.

3. Pour in a splash of dry sherry to deglaze the pan.

4. Pour in the chicken bone broth and bring to a boil. Stir in the tomatoes and bay laurel. Season with salt and pepper to taste. Turn the heat to medium-low and continue to cook 10 minutes longer.

5. Add the reserved pork back to the pot, partially cover, and continue to simmer for 45 minutes longer. Garnish with cilantro and serve hot. Bon appétit!

Nutrition:

Calories: 332 fat: 15g protein: 41g carbs: 4g net carbs: 3g fiber: 1g

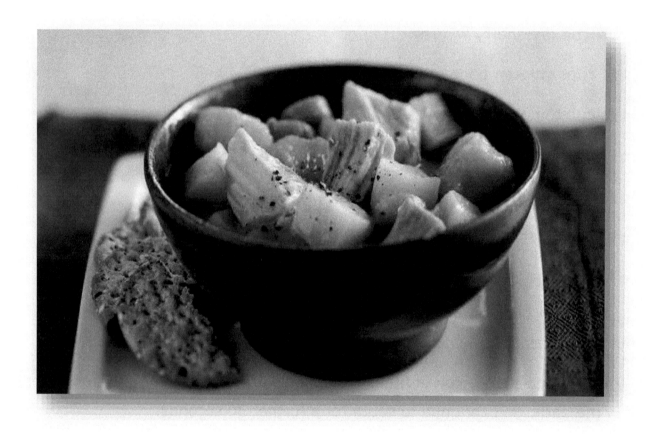

Chapter 2. Mains

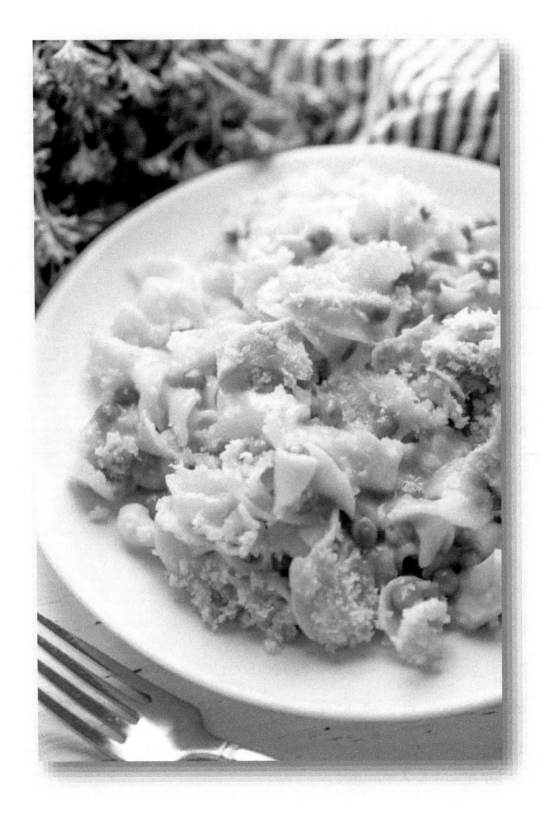

9. Turkey Chili

Preparation time: 15 minutes

Cooking time: 120 minutes

Servings: 8

Ingredients:

- 2 tablespoons of olive oil
- 1 small yellow onion, chopped
- 1 green bell pepper, seeded and chopped
- 4 garlic cloves, minced
- 1 jalapeño pepper, chopped
- 1 teaspoon of dried thyme, crushed
- 2 tablespoons of red chili powder
- 1 tablespoon of ground cumin
- 2 pounds of lean ground turkey
- 2 cups of fresh tomatoes, chopped finely
- 2 ounces of sugar-free tomato paste
- 2 cups of homemade chicken broth
- 1 cup of water
- Salt and ground black pepper, as required
- 1 cup of cheddar cheese, shredded Directions:

1. In a large Dutch oven, heat oil over medium heat and sauté the onion and bell pepper for about 5-7 minutes.

2. Add the garlic, jalapeño pepper, thyme, and spices and sauté for about 1 minute.

3. Add the turkey and cook for about 4-5 minutes.

4. Stir in the tomatoes, tomato paste, and cacao powder, and cook for about 2 minutes.

5. Add in the broth and water and bring to a boil.

6. Now, reduce the heat to low and simmer, covered for about 2 hours.

7. Add in salt and black pepper and remove from the heat.

8. Top with cheddar cheese and serve hot.

Nutrition: Calories: 308 Cal, Fat: 20g, Carbs: 10g, Protein: 8g, Fiber: 3g.

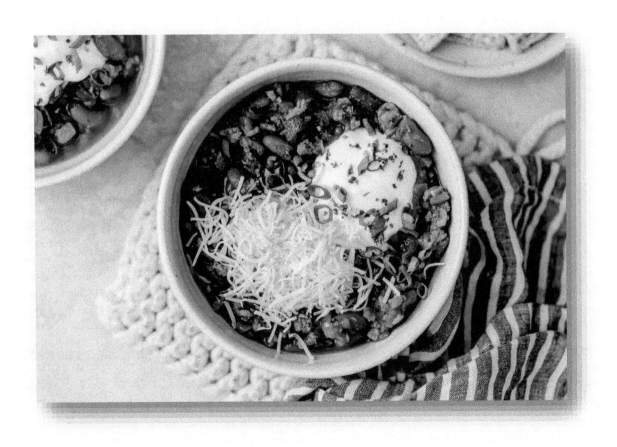

10. Keto Wraps with Cream Cheese and Salmon

Preparation time: 5 minutes

Cooking time: 10 minutes

Servings: 2

Ingredients:

- 80g of cream cheese
- 1 tablespoon of dill or other fresh herbs
- 30g of smoked salmon
- 1 egg
- 15g of butter
- Pinch of cayenne pepper
- Pepper and salt Directions:

1. Beat the egg well in a bowl. With 1 egg, you can make two thin wraps in a small frying pan.

2. Melt the butter over medium heat in a small frying pan. Once the butter has melted, add half of the beaten egg to the pan. Move the pan back and forth so that the entire bottom is covered with a very thin layer of egg. Turn down the heat!

3. Carefully loosen the egg on the edges with a silicone spatula and turn the wafer-thin omelet as soon as the egg is no longer dripping (about 45 seconds to 1 minute). You can do this by sliding it onto a lid or plate and then sliding it back into the pan. Let the other side be cooked for about 30 seconds and then remove from the pan. The omelet must be nice and light yellow. Repeat for the rest of the beaten egg.

4. Once the omelets are ready, let them cool on a cutting board or plate and make the filling. Cut the dill into small pieces and put them in a bowl.

5. Add the cream cheese and the salmon, cut into small pieces. Mix. Add a tiny bit of cayenne pepper and mix well. Taste immediately, and then season with salt and pepper.

6. Spread a layer on the wrap and roll it up. Cut the wrap in half and keep it in the fridge until you are ready to eat it. Nutrition: Calories: 237, Carbohydrates: 14.7g, Protein: 15g, Fat: 5g.

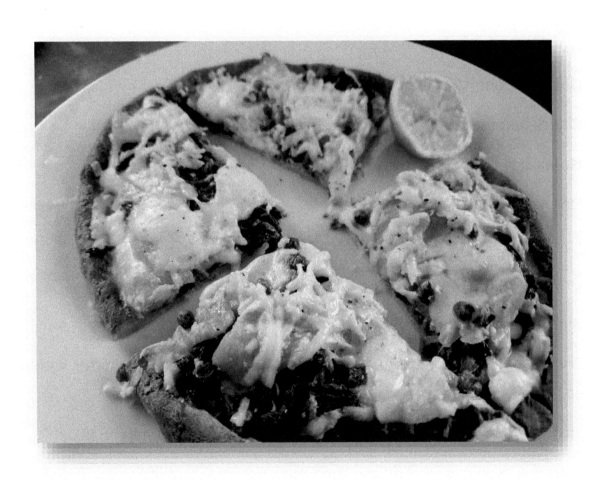

11. Tuna Casserole

Preparation time: 15 minutes

Cooking time: 10 minutes

Servings: 4

Ingredients:

- Sixteen ounces of tuna in oil
- Two tablespoons of butter
- Salt
- Black pepper
- One teaspoon of chili powder
- Celery, six stalks
- Green bell pepper, one
- One yellow onion
- Four ounces of parmesan cheese, grated
- One cup of mayonnaise Directions:

1. Warm-up oven to 400°F.

2. Fry the onion, bell pepper, and celery chops in the melted butter within five minutes.

3. Mix with the chili powder, parmesan cheese, tuna, and mayonnaise.

4. Grease a baking pan. Add the tuna mixture into the fried vegetables.

5. Bake within twenty minutes. Serve. Nutrition: Calories 953, Net carbs 5g, Fat 83g, Protein 43g.

12. Keto Red Curry

Preparation time: 20 minutes

Cooking time: 15-20 min

Servings: 6

Ingredients:

- 1 cup of broccoli florets
- 1 large handful of fresh spinach
- 4 tbsp. of coconut oil
- 1/4 medium onion
- 1 tsp. of garlic, minced
- 1 tsp. of fresh ginger, peeled and minced
- 2 tsp. of soy sauce
- 1 tbsp. of red curry paste
- 1/2 cup of coconut cream

Directions:

1. Add half the coconut oil to a saucepan and heat over medium-high heat.

2. When the oil is hot, put the onion in the pan and sauté for 3-4 minutes, until it is semi-translucent.

3. Sauté garlic, stirring, just until fragrant, about 30 seconds.

4. Lower the heat to medium-low and add broccoli florets. Sauté, stirring, for about 1-2 minutes.

5. Now, add the red curry paste. Sauté until the paste is fragrant, then mix everything.

6. Add the spinach on top of the vegetable mixture. When the spinach begins to wilt, add the coconut cream and stir.

7. Add the rest of the coconut oil, the soy sauce, and the minced ginger. Bring to a simmer for 5-10 minutes. Serve hot. Nutrition: Calories: 265, Fat: 7.1g, Fiber: 6.9g, Carbohydrates: 2.1g, Protein: 4.4g.

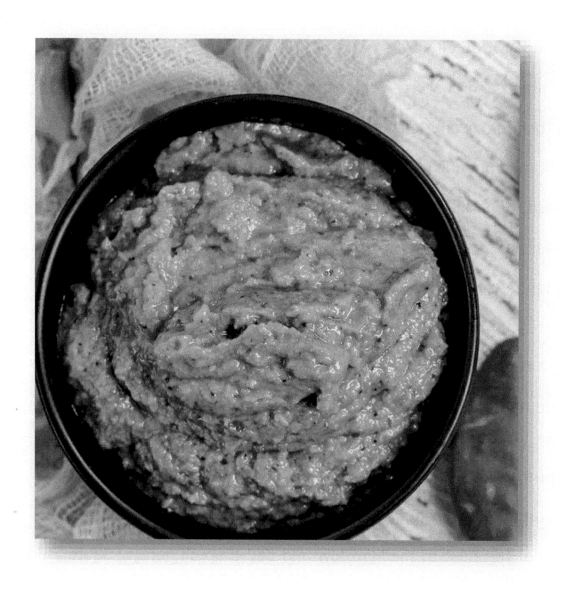

Chapter 3. Sides

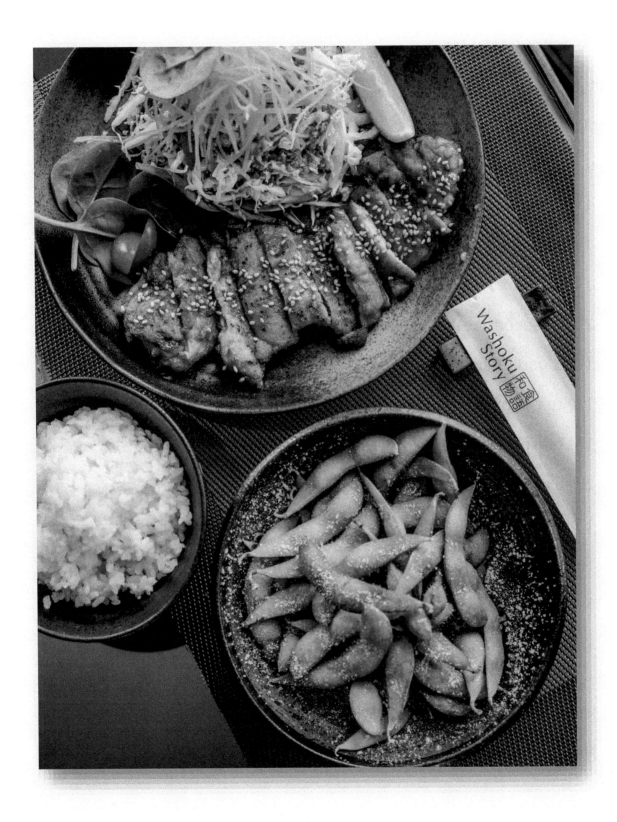

13. Creamy Kale Salad

Preparation Time: 15 minutes

Cooking Time: 0 minutes

Servings: 3

Ingredients:

- 1 bunch spinach
- 1 1/2 tablespoon lemon juice
- 1 cup sour cream
- 1 cup roasted macadamia
- 2 tablespoons sesame seeds oil
- 1 1/2 garlic clove, minced
- 1/2 teaspoon black pepper
- 1/4 teaspoon salt
- 2 tablespoons lime juice
- 1 bunch kale
- Toppings:
- 1 1/2 Avocado, diced
- 1/4 cup Pecans, chopped Directions:

1. First of all, please confirm you've all the ingredients out there. Chop kale and wash kale then remove the ribs.

2. Now transfer kale to a large bowl.

3. One thing remains to be done. Add sour cream, lime juice, macadamia, sesame seeds oil, pepper, salt, garlic.

4. Finally, mix thoroughly. Top with your avocado and pecans. Serve& enjoy.

Nutrition:

Calories: 291 Fat: 5.1g Fiber: 12.9g

Carbohydrates: 4.3 g Protein: 11.8g

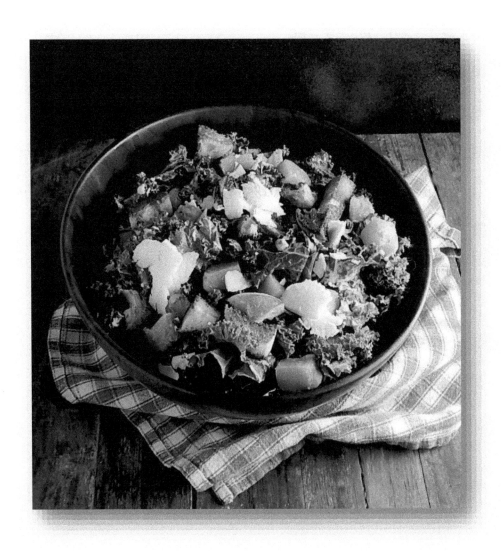

14. Brussels sprouts with Bacon

Preparation Time: 5 minutes

Cooking Time: 40 minutes

Servings: 6

Ingredients:

- 16 ounces Brussels sprouts
- 1 teaspoon salt
- 16 ounces bacon, pasteurized
- 2/3 teaspoon ground black pepper Directions:

1. Preheat oven to 400ºF.

2. Slice every sprout in half and then slice bacon lengthwise into small pieces.

3. Take a baking sheet, line it with parchment paper, spread Brussels sprouts halves and bacon on it, and then season with salt and black pepper.

4. Bake for 35–40 minutes until sprouts turn golden-brown, and bacon is crisp.

5. Serve straight away. Nutrition:

Calories: 101 Fat: 5.1g Fiber: 10g

Carbohydrates: 1 g Protein: 5.5g

15. Bacon Mashed Cauliflower

Preparation Time: 15 Minutes

Cooking Time: 16 Minutes

Servings: 6

Ingredients:

- 6 slices bacon
- 3 heads cauliflower, leaves removed
- 2 cups water
- 2 tbsps. Melted butter
- ½ cup buttermilk
- Salt and black pepper to taste
- ¼ cup grated yellow cheddar cheese
- 2 tbsps. Chopped chives

Directions:

1. Preheat oven to 350ºF. Cook bacon in a heated skillet over medium heat for 5 minutes until crispy. Remove to a paper towel-lined plate, allow to cool, and crumble. Set aside and keep bacon fat. Boil cauli heads in water in a pot over high heat for 7 minutes, until tender. Drain and put in a bowl.

2. Include butter, buttermilk, salt, black pepper, and puree using a hand blender until smooth and creamy. Lightly grease a casserole dish with the bacon fat and spread the mash on it.

3. Sprinkle with cheddar cheese and place under the broiler for 4 minutes on high until the cheese melts. Remove and top with bacon and chopped chives. Serve with pan-seared scallops.

Nutrition:

Kcal 312 Fat 25g

Net Carbs 6g Protein 14g

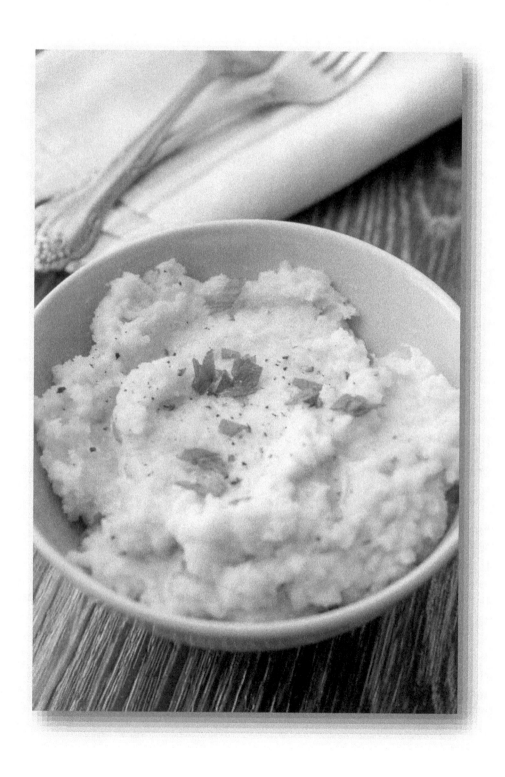

16. Grilled Mediterranean Veggies

Preparation Time: 10 minutes

Cooking Time: 15 minutes

Servings: 4

Ingredients:

- 1/4 cup (56 g/2 oz) ghee or butter
- 2 small (200 g/7.1 oz) red, orange, or yellow peppers
- 3 medium (600 g/21.2 oz) zucchini
- 1 medium (500 g/17.6 oz) eggplant
- 1 medium (100 g/3.5 oz) red onion

Directions:

1. Set the oven to broil to the highest setting.
2. In a small bowl, mix the melted ghee and crushed garlic.
3. Wash all the vegetables.
4. Halve, deseed, and slice the bell peppers into strips.
5. Slice the zucchini widthwise into 1/4-inch (about 1/2 cm) pieces.
6. Wash the eggplant and slice.
7. Quarter each slice into 1/4-inch (about 1/2 cm) pieces.
8. Peel and slice the onion into medium wedges and separate the sections using your hands.
9. Place the vegetables in a bowl and add the chopped herbs, ghee with garlic, salt, and black pepper. The vegetables must be spread on a baking sheet, ideally on a roasting rack or net, so that the vegetables don't become soggy from the juices.

10. Put it in the oven and let it cook for about 15 minutes.

11. Be careful not to burn them.

12. When done, the vegetables should be slightly tender but still crisp.

13. Serve with meat dishes or bake with cheese such as feta, mozzarella, or Halloumi.

Nutrition:

Calories: 176 Fat: 4.5g Fiber: 9.3g

Carbohydrates: 3.1g Protein: 5.2 g

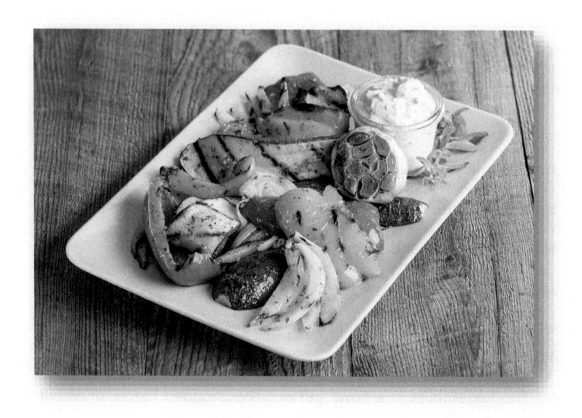

17. BLT Salad Preparation

Time: 15 minutes

Cooking Time: 0 minutes

Servings: 4

Ingredients:

- 2 tablespoons melted bacon fat
- 2 tablespoons red wine vinegar
- Freshly ground black pepper
- 4 cups shredded lettuce
- 1 tomato, chopped
- 6 bacon slices, cooked and chopped
- 2 hardboiled eggs, chopped
- 1 tablespoon roasted unsalted sunflower seeds
- 1 teaspoon toasted sesame seeds
- 1 cooked chicken breast, sliced (optional)

Directions:

1. In a medium bowl, whisk together the bacon fat and vinegar until emulsified. Season with black pepper.

2. Add the tomato and lettuce to the bowl and toss the vegetables with the dressing.

3. Divide the salad between 4 plates and top each with equal amounts of bacon, egg, sunflower seeds, sesame seeds, and chicken (if using). Serve. Nutrition:

Calories: 287 Fat: 9.4g Fiber: 11g

Carbohydrates: 3.8 g Protein: 9.9g

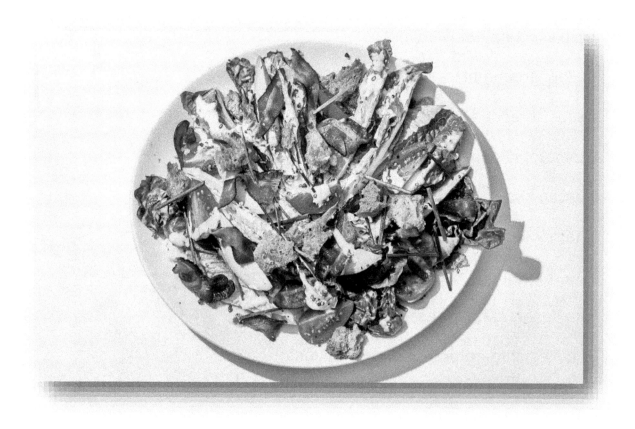

18. Crab Cakes with Almond Flour

Preparation time: 1 hour 10 minutes

Cooking time: 15 minutes

Servings: 4 Ingredients:

- 8 oz fresh crab meat, shells removed
- 1 Tbsp garlic, minced
- ¼ cup parsley, chopped
- 1 egg, slightly beaten
- 1 Tbsp avocado oil mayonnaise
- 1 Tbsp mustard
- ½ tsp kosher salt
- ½ tsp dried thyme
- 1/8 tsp cayenne pepper
- ½ cup almond flour
- 2 Tbsp butter, for frying Directions:

1. In a separate bowl, combine the crabmeat, garlic, parsley, egg, mayonnaise, mustard, kosher salt, thyme, cayenne pepper, and almond flour. Stir well. Form 4 cakes and place them into a fridge for 1 hour.

2. Melt the butter in the pan and put in your crab cakes. Fry for about 5-7 minutes on each side.

Nutrition: Carbohydrates – 4 g

Fat – 17 g Protein – 13 g Calories – 219

Chapter 4. Seafood

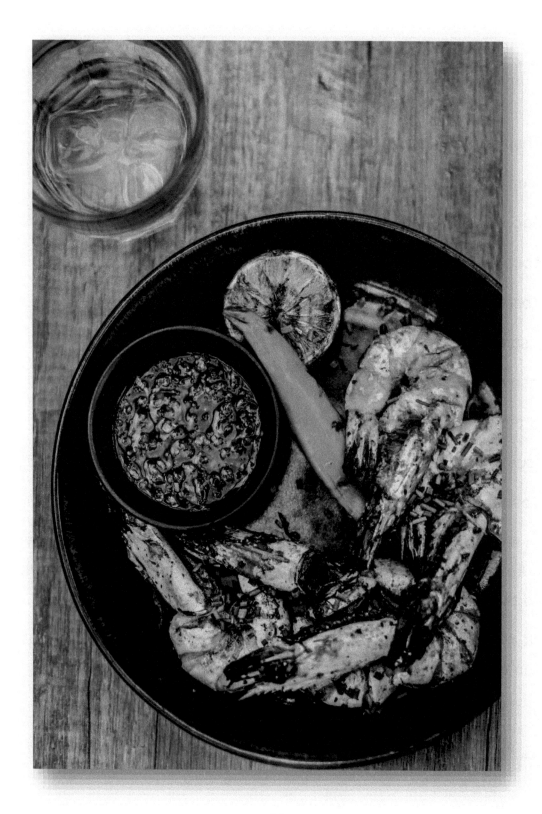

19. Quick Butter Cod

Preparation Time: 10 minutes

Cooking Time: 5 minutes

Servings: 4 Ingredients:

- 1 ½ lbs. cod fillets, cut into pieces
- ½ tsp paprika
- ¼ tsp ground pepper
- ¼ tsp garlic powder
- 6 tbsp. butter
- ½ tsp salt Directions:

1. On a small bowl, mix paprika, pepper, garlic powder, and salt.
2. Coat fish pieces with seasoning mixture.
3. Melt 2 tbsp. of butter during a large pan over medium-high heat.
4. Add fish pieces to the pan and cook for two minutes.
5. Turn heat to medium. Add remaining butter on top of fish pieces and cook for 3-4 minutes.
6. Once fish is cooked thoroughly, then remove the pan from heat.
7. Add juice and stir well.
8. Serve and luxuriate in. Nutrition:

Calories: 291 Fat: 18.8g

Carbohydrates: 0.4g Sugar: 0.1g

Protein: 30.6g Cholesterol: 129mg

20. Creamy Mackerel

Preparation Time: 10 minutes

Cooking Time: 20 minutes

Servings: 4

Ingredients:

- 2 shallots, minced
- 2 spring onions, chopped
- 2 tablespoons olive oil
- 4 mackerel fillets, skinless and cut into medium cubes
- 1 cup heavy cream
- 1 teaspoon cumin, ground
- ½ teaspoon oregano, dried
- A pinch of salt and black pepper
- 2 tablespoons chives, chopped Directions:

1. Heat a pan with the oil over medium heat, add the spring onions and the shallots, stir and sauté for 5 minutes.

2. Add the fish and cook it for 4 minutes.

3. Add the rest of the ingredients, bring to a simmer, cook everything for 10 minutes more, divide between plates, and serve.

Nutrition:

Calories: 403 Fat: 33.9g Fiber: 0.4g Carbs: 2.7g Protein: 22g

21. Herb Crusted Tilapia

Preparation Time: 5 minutes

Cooking Time: 10 minutes

Servings: 2

Ingredients

- 2 fillets of tilapia
- ½ tsp garlic powder
- ½ tsp Italian seasoning
- ½ tsp dried parsley
- 1/3 tsp salt Seasoning:
- 2 tbsp. melted butter, unsalted
- 1 tbsp. avocado oil Directions:

1. Turn on the broiler and then let it preheat.

2. Meanwhile, take a small bowl, place melted butter in it, stir in oil and garlic powder until mixed, and then brush this mixture over tilapia fillets.

3. Stir together remaining spices and then sprinkle them generously on tilapia until well coated.

4. Place seasoned tilapia in a baking pan, place the pan under the broiler and then bake for 10 minutes until tender and golden, brushing with garlic-butter every 2 minutes.

5. Serve.

Nutrition: 520 Calories; 35 g Fats; 36.2 g Protein; 13.6 g Net Carb; 0.6 g Fiber;

22. Shrimp Avocado Salad

Preparation Time: 10 minutes

Cooking Time: 5 minutes

Servings: 4 Ingredients:

- 16 oz. shrimp, thawed and drained
- 1 avocado, pitted and diced
- ¼ cup celery, chopped
- 1 small onion, chopped
- 2½ tbsp. fresh dill, chopped
- 1 tbsp. vinegar
- 1 tsp Dijon mustard
- ½ cup mayonnaise
- Pepper Salt Directions:

1. On a small bowl, mix mayonnaise, dill, vinegar, and mustard. Set aside.
2. Add shrimp, onion, and celery during a bowl.
3. Pour mayonnaise mixture over shrimp and stir well.
4. Cover and place within the refrigerator for 1-2 hours.
5. Add avocado and serve immediately.

Nutrition:

Calories: 279 Fat: 13.1g

Carbohydrates: 12.5g Sugar: 2.7g

Protein: 27g Cholesterol: 246mg

Chapter 5. Poultry

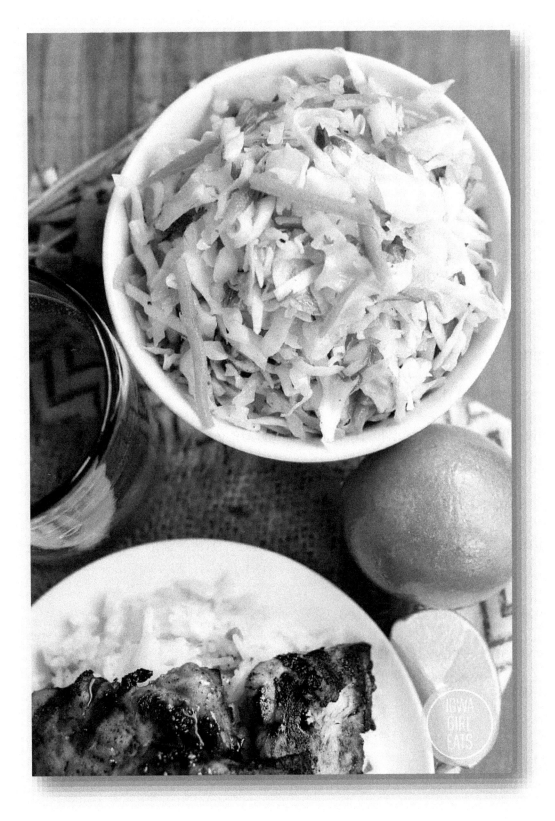

23. Parmesan Chicken

Preparation Time: 10 minutes

Cooking Time: 35 minutes

Servings: 4

Ingredients:

- 1 lb. chicken breasts, skinless and boneless
- 1/2 cup parmesan cheese, grated
- 3/4 cup mayonnaise
- 1 tsp garlic powder
- 1/2 tsp Italian seasoning Directions:

1. Preheat the oven to 375 F.
2. Spray baking dish with cooking spray.
3. Now, in a small bowl, mix together mayonnaise, garlic powder, poultry seasoning, and pepper.
4. Place chicken breasts into the prepared baking dish.
5. Spread mayonnaise mixture over chicken, then sprinkles cheese on top of chicken.
6. Bake chicken for 35 minutes.
7. Serve and enjoy. Nutrition:

Calories 391

Fat 23 g

Carbohydrates 11 g

Sugar 3 g

Protein 33 g

Cholesterol 112 mg

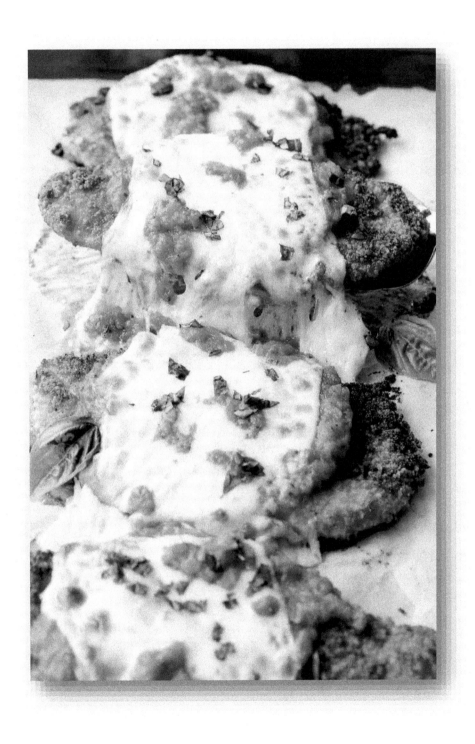

24. Chili Lime Chicken with Coleslaw

Preparation time: 35 minutes

Cooking time: 8 minutes

Servings: 2

Ingredients:

- 1 chicken thigh, boneless
- 2 ounces coleslaw
- ¼ teaspoon minced garlic
- ¾ tablespoon apple cider vinegar
- ½ of a lime, juiced, zested
- ¼ teaspoon paprika
- ¼ teaspoon salt
- 2 tablespoons avocado oil
- 1 tablespoon unsalted butter Directions:

1. Prepare the marinade and for this, take a medium bowl, add vinegar, oil, garlic, paprika, salt, lime juice, and zest and stir until well mixed.

2. Cut chicken thighs into bite-size pieces, toss until well mixed, and marinate it in the refrigerator for 30 minutes.

3. Then take a skillet pan, place it over medium-high heat, add butter and marinated chicken pieces and cook for 8 minutes until golden brown and thoroughly cooked.

4. Serve chicken with coleslaw. Nutrition:

Calories: 157.3 Fat: 12.8g Protein: 9g Carbs: 1g Fiber: 0.5g

25. Lemongrass Chicken

Preparation Time: 10 minutes

Cooking Time: 15 minutes

Servings: 4

Ingredients:

- 4 chicken thighs, bone-in
- 2 tbsp. brown sugar
- 3 tbsp. sugar
- 2 tbsp. fresh lime juice
- 3 tbsp. soy sauce
- 3 tbsp. fish sauce
- 1 tbsp. ginger, sliced
- 1 shallot, sliced
- 1 tbsp. garlic, chopped
- 2 lemongrass stalks, sliced
- 2 tbsp. water
- 1 1/2 tbsp. cornstarch Directions:

1. In a mixing bowl, mix together chicken, 3 tbsp. Water, soy sauce, fish sauce, lime juice, brown sugar, lemongrass, ginger, shallot, and garlic. Cover & place in the refrigerator for 1 hour.

2. Place marinated chicken into the instant pot.

3. Seal pot with lid & cook on high pressure for 7 minutes.

4. When done, allow releasing pressure naturally for 10 mins. Then release the remaining pressure using quick release. Remove lid.

5. Remove chicken from pot and set aside.

6. Mix together cornstarch and 2 tbsp. Water and pour into the instant pot and cook on sauté mode until sauce thickens.

7. Pour sauce over chicken and coat well. Clean the instant pot.

8. Place chicken in instant pot air fryer basket and place basket in the pot.

9. Seal pot w/ air fryer lid & select broil mode & set timer for 5 minutes.

10. Serve and enjoy. Nutrition:

Calories 374

Fat 19 g

Carbohydrates 25 g

Sugar 15 g

Protein 43 g

Cholesterol 130 mg

26. Crispy Crust Whole Chicken

Preparation Time: 10 minutes

Cooking Time: 45 minutes

Servings: 4

Ingredients:

- 1 whole chicken
- 1 1/2 cups chicken broth
- 2 tbsp. Montreal steak seasoning
- 1 tsp Italian seasoning
- 1 tsp paprika
- 1 tsp onion powder
- 1 tsp garlic powder
- 2 tbsp. olive oil

Directions:

1. Pour broth into the instant pot.

2. Mix together Montreal steak seasoning, Italian seasoning, paprika, onion powder, and garlic powder.

3. Brush chicken with olive oil & rub with seasoning. Place chicken in the air fryer basket and place basket in the instant pot.

4. Seal the pot with pressure cooking lid and cook on high pressure for 25 minutes.

5. When done, allow releasing pressure naturally for 15 minutes then release the remaining pressure using quick release. Remove lid.

6. Remove liquid from the instant pot.

7. Seal pot w/ air fryer lid and select air fry mode & set the temperature to 400 F and timer for 10 minutes.

8. Turn chicken to the other side and air fry for 10 minutes more.

9. Serve and enjoy. Nutrition:

Calories 925

Fat 44 g

Carbohydrates 8 g

Sugar 8 g

Protein 127 g

Cholesterol 390 mg

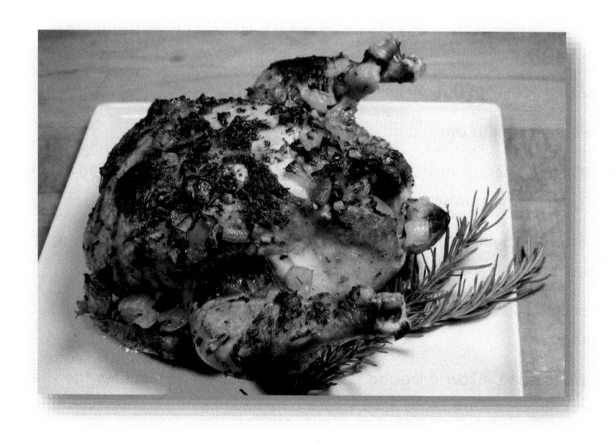

Chapter 6. Meat

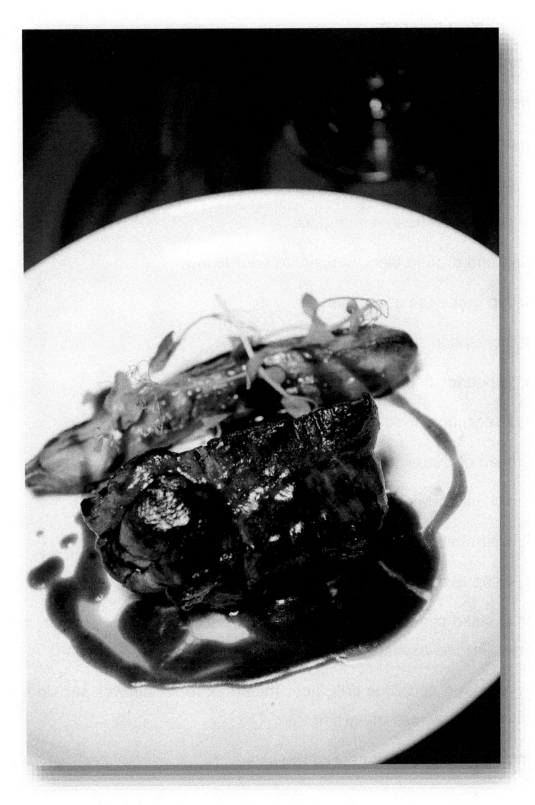

27. Greek-Style Cold Beef Salad

Preparation Time: 15 minutes

Cooking Time: 5 minutes

Servings: 6

Ingredients

- 1 orange bell pepper, thinly sliced
- 1 green bell pepper, thinly sliced
- 1 tablespoon fresh lemon juice
- Salt and ground black pepper, to your liking
- 1 cup grape tomatoes, halved
- 1 tablespoon soy sauce
- 1 ½ pounds beef rump steak
- 1/2 teaspoon dried oregano
- 1 head of butter lettuce, leaves separated
- 1 red onion, peeled and thinly sliced
- 2 cucumbers, thinly sliced
- 1/4 cup extra-virgin olive oil Directions:

1. In a salad container, toss the onions, cucumbers, and tomato, bell pepper, and butter lettuce leaves.

2. Fore heat a barbecue grill; heat the steak for 3 minutes per side. After that, thinly slice steak across the grain.

3. Include the slices of meat to the salad.

4. Prepare the dressing by whisking the oregano, salt, pepper, lemon juice, olive oil and soy sauce.

5. Dress the salad and enjoy well- chilled.

Nutrition: Calories 315, Protein 37.5g, Fat 13.8g, Carbs 6.4g, Sugar 2.4g

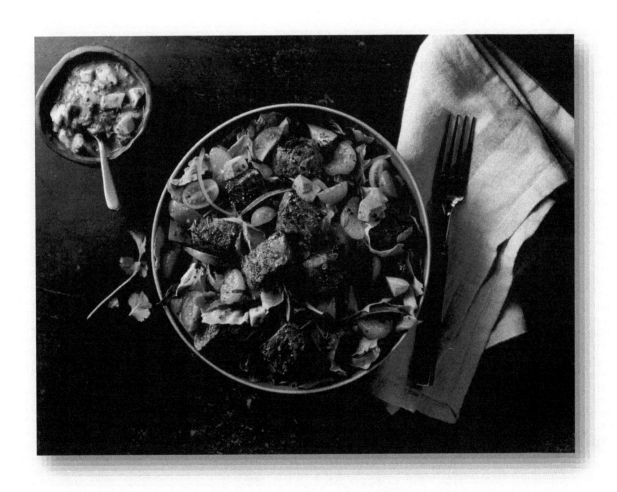

28. Beef Wellington

Preparation time: 20 minutes

Cooking time: 40 minutes

Servings: 4

Ingredients

- 2 (4-ounce) grass-fed beef tenderloin steaks, halved
- Salt and ground black pepper, as required
- 1 tablespoon butter
- 1 cup mozzarella cheese, shredded
- ½ cup almond flour
- 4 tablespoons liver pate

Directions:

1. Preheat your oven to 400°F.
2. Grease a baking sheet.
3. Season the steaks with salt and black pepper evenly.
4. In a frying pan, melt the butter over medium-high heat and sear the beef steaks for about 2–3 minutes per side.
5. Remove frying pan from the heat and set aside to cool completely.
6. In a microwave-safe bowl, add the mozzarella cheese and microwave for about 1 minute.
7. Remove from the microwave and immediately, stir in the almond flour until a dough form.
8. Place the dough between 2 parchment paper pieces and with a rolling pin, roll to flatten it.

9. Remove the upper parchment paper piece.

10. Divide the rolled dough into 4 pieces.

11. Place 1 tablespoon of pate onto each dough piece and top with 1 steak piece.

12. Cover each steak piece with dough completely.

13. Arrange the covered steak pieces onto the prepared baking sheet in a single layer.

14. Bake for about 20–30 minutes or until the pastry is a golden-brown.

15. Serve warm. Nutrition:

Calories 545 Net Carbs 3.9 g Total Fat 36.6 g

Saturated Fat 11.3 g Cholesterol 190 mg

Sodium 459 mg Total Carbs 6.9 g Fiber 3 g

Sugar 1 g

Protein 48.2 g

29. Oven Roasted Rib-Eye Steak

Preparation Time: 10 minutes

Cooking Time: 25 minutes

Servings: 6

Ingredients

- 1 teaspoon sea salt
- 1 tablespoon olive oil
- 1/2 teaspoon ground black pepper
- 2 tablespoons apple cider vinegar
- 1 ½ pounds rib-eye steak
- 2 garlic cloves, minced
- 1/2 cup Worcester sauce

Directions:

1. Preheat your oven to 3500F. Lubricate a roasting pan with a nonstick cooking spray.

2. Heat olive oil in a skillet that is forehead over medium-high heat. Season the steak using salt and black pepper; sear the steak until just browned or duration of about 3 minutes.

3. Put the steak in the prepared roasting pan. In a mixing container, merge the Worcester sauce, garlic and apple cider vinegar. Transfer this mixture over the steak.

4. Now, shut tightly with a piece of foil. Roast the steak for about 20 minutes or until it becomes tender and well browned. Enjoy!

Nutrition: Calories 343, Protein 20.1g, Fat 27.3g, Carbs 3g, Sugar 0g

30. Stuffed Tomatoes with Cotija Cheese

Preparation Time: 5 minutes

Cooking Time: 30 minutes

Servings: 4

Ingredients

- 1 cup scallions, chopped
- 2 tablespoons tomato paste, sugar- free
- 1/2 teaspoon cumin seeds
- 2 cloves garlic, minced
- 1 teaspoon mild paprika
- 1-pound ground beef
- 1 tablespoon olive oil
- Salt and pepper, to your liking
- 1/2 cup beef broth
- 1 teaspoon dried coriander leaves
- 8 tomatoes, scoop out the pulp and chop it
- 3/4 cup Cotija cheese, shredded Directions:

1. Begin by preheating your oven to 3500F. Softly grease a casserole dish with a cooking spray.

2. Apply heat to the oil in a saucepan over moderately high heat. Sauté the scallions and garlic till they become aromatic.

3. Stir in ground meat; cook for 5 minutes, crumbling with a spatula. Include tomato paste and heat until heated thoroughly. Season with pepper, salt, and cumin seeds.

4. Fill the tomatoes with beef mixture and move them to the already prepared casserole dish.

5. In a mixing container, whisk tomato pulp with coriander, paprika and broth. Transfer the mixture over the stuffed tomatoes.

6. Bake until tomatoes become tender, for about 20 minutes. Top with Cotija cheese and bake an additional time of 5 minutes. Bon appétit!

Nutrition: Calories 244, Protein 28.9g, Fat 9.6g, Carbs 6g, Sugar 4g

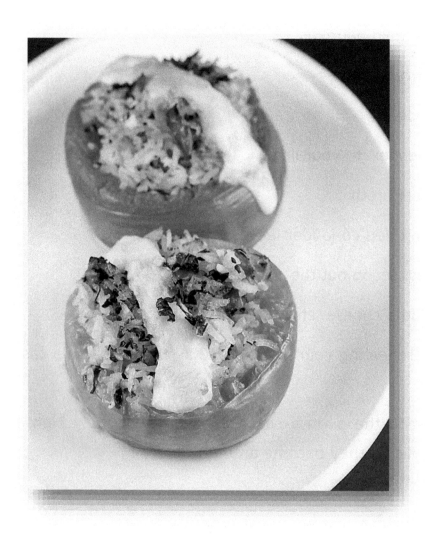

31. Coconut Fajita Chicken

Preparation time: 10 minutes

Cooking time: 1 hour 10 minutes

Servings: 4 Ingredients:

- 4 boneless, skinless chicken breasts
- ½ white onion, peeled and thinly chopped
- 1 red bell pepper, seeded and chopped
- 1 yellow bell pepper, seeded and chopped
- 1 green bell pepper, seeded and chopped
- ½ can full-fat coconut milk
- 1 Tbsp coconut oil
- 1 pinch red pepper flakes Directions:

1. Preheat your oven to 425°F, and coat a baking dish with coconut oil.

2. In a large skillet, sauté the chicken with the onion and bell peppers until the chicken and vegetables begin to brown.

3. Add the coconut milk and stir.

4. Transfer the chicken mixture into the baking dish and bake for about 45 minutes.

5. Season with red pepper flakes. Nutrition:

Carbohydrates – 5 g Fat – 14 g

Protein – 27 g Calories – 251

Chapter 7. Vegetables

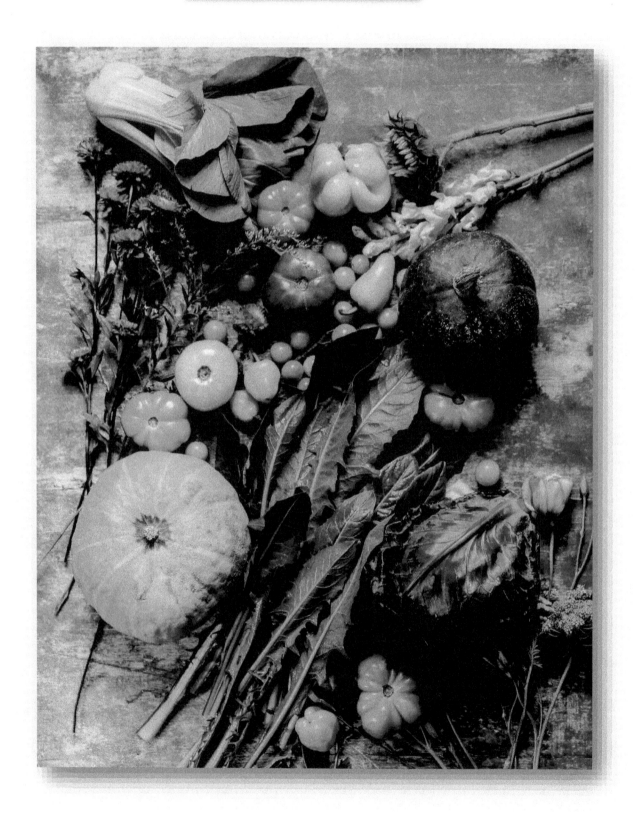

32. Low-carb cheesy omelet

Preparation Time: 5 minutes

Cooking time: 10 minutes

Servings: 2 Ingredients:

- 6 eggs
- 7 ounces (198 g) shredded Cheddar cheese
- Salt and ground black pepper, to taste
- 3 ounces (85 g) butter Directions:

1. In a bowl, whisk all the eggs until they are frothy and smooth. Add half of the Cheddar and blend well.

2. Add the pepper and salt to season.

3. In a frying pan, melt the butter over medium-high heat, then pour the egg mixture and cook for a few minutes until you see the eggs at the edges of the pan beginning to set.

4. Reduce the heat to low as you continue cooking the mixture for 3 minutes until it is almost cooked. Flip the omelet halfway through the cooking time. Scatter the remaining cheese on top and cook for another 1 to 2 minutes until the cheese melts.

5. Fold your omelet and serve while warm.

6. STORAGE: Store in an airtight container in the fridge for up to 4 days or in the freezer for up to one month.

7. REHEAT: Microwave, covered, until the desired temperature is reached or reheat in a frying pan or air fryer / instant pot, covered, on medium.

8. SERVE IT WITH: To make this a complete meal, serve the omelet with a tomato salad or avocado sticks. Nutrition:

Calories: 899 Total

Fat 79g Fiber: 0g

Net carbs: 5g Protein: 39.2g

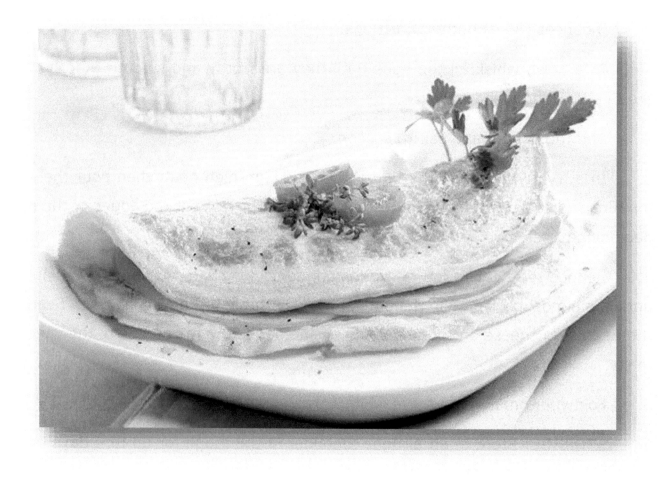

33. Margherita Mushroom Pizza

Preparation time: 15 minutes

Cooking time: 15 minutes

Servings: 6

Ingredient:

- 6 large portobello mushrooms, stems removed
- 1 teaspoon garlic, minced
- 1 cup sugar-free tomato sauce
- 2 cups Mozzarella cheese, shredded
- 2 tablespoons chopped fresh basil, for garnish
- ½ cup extra-virgin olive oil

Directions:

1. Preheat the oven to 350°F (180°C), and line a baking tray with aluminum foil. Set aside.

2. Combine the mushrooms, garlic, and olive oil in a medium bowl. Toss well until the mushrooms are fully coated.

3. Arrange the mushrooms (gill-side down) on the baking tray. Roast in the preheated oven for about 12 minutes, flipping once, or until the mushrooms are firm but tender.

4. Remove from the oven and pour the tomato sauce over the mushroom caps. Sprinkle the Mozzarella cheese on top.

5. Return the baking tray to the oven and roast for 1 to 2 minutes more, or until the cheese melts.

6. Remove from the oven and garnish with the chopped basil.

TIP: To add a good dose of fat and flavor, you can sprinkle the chopped Italian sausage or prosciutto on top of the mushrooms other than Mozzarella cheese. Nutrition:

Calories: 317 fat: 25.3g protein: 16.2g net carbs: 6.1g fiber: 3g

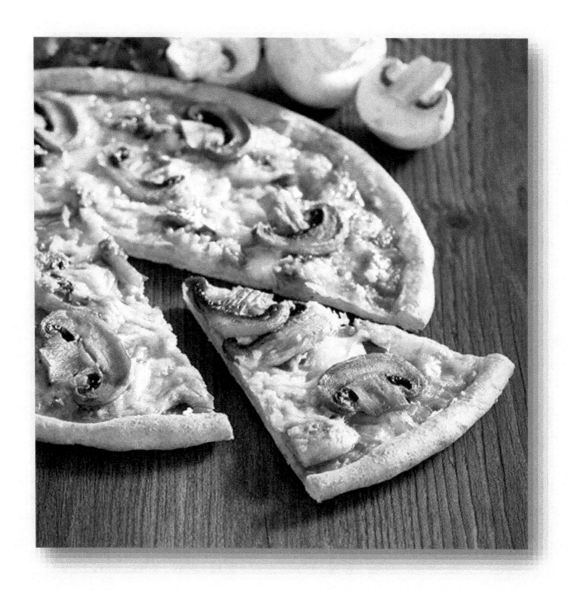

34. Cauliflower, leeks and broccoli

Preparation Time: 5 minutes

Cooking time: 15 minutes

Servings: 4

You will enjoy the cheesy cauliflower that will incorporate the healthy broccoli. It is an easy-to-prepare recipe. This recipe is rich in nutrients with low carbohydrates. The inclusion of thyme makes the flavor wonderful.

Ingredients:

- 8 ounces (227 g) cauliflower, chopped in bite-sized pieces
- 3 ounces (85 g) leeks, chopped in bite-sized pieces
- 1-pound (454 g) broccoli, chopped in bite-sized pieces
- 3 ounces (85 g) butter
- 5 ounces (142 g) shredded cheese
- ½ cup fresh thyme
- 4 tablespoons sour cream
- Pepper and salt to taste Directions:

1. In a skillet over medium-high heat, add butter and heat to melt. Add the leeks, broccoli and cauliflower. Fry the vegetables until they become golden brown.

2. Add the cheese, thyme and sour cream. Stir well until the cheese melts. Add pepper and salt for seasoning.

3. Transfer them to a platter. Allow to cool for a few minutes before serving

4. STORAGE: Store in an airtight container in the fridge for up to 4 days or in the freezer for up to one month.

5. REHEAT: Microwave, covered, until the desired temperature is reached or reheat in a frying pan or air fryer / instant pot, covered, on medium.

6. SERVE IT WITH: To make this a complete meal, serve with mushroom pork chops.

Nutrition:

Calories: 368 Total

Fat 32g Fiber: 5.4g

Net carbs: 9.3g Protein: 14.2g

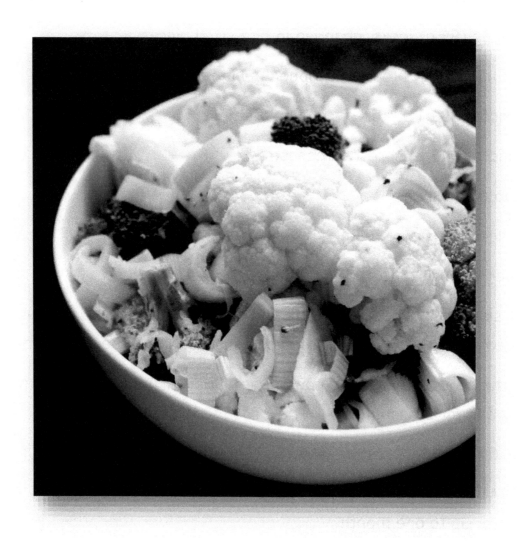

35. Braised Fennel with Lemon

Preparation time: 10 minutes

Cooking time: 1 hour and 40 minutes

Servings: 2

Ingredients:

- 2 pounds fennel bulbs
- ¾ pound lemons
- 1 teaspoon minced garlic
- 1 ½ teaspoon sea salt
- ¾ teaspoon cracked black pepper
- 2 teaspoons fresh rosemary, chopped
- 1 teaspoon fresh thyme, chopped
- 6 tablespoons apple cider vinegar
- 1/4 cup olive oil

Directions:

1. Set oven to 375 degrees F and let preheat.
2. In the meantime, slice fennel bulb into wedges, slice lemons into thin wedges and arrange in a large baking dish in a single layer.
3. Whisk together garlic, rosemary, thyme, vinegar, and oil until combined, pour this mixture evenly over vegetables in the baking dish, season with salt and black pepper and cover with aluminum foil.
4. Place this baking dish into the heated oven and bake for 1 hour, then uncover baking dish and continue baking for 30 to 40 minutes or until vegetables are roasted and crispy.

5. Serve straight away with baked chicken.

Nutrition:

Calories: 128 Cal, Carbs: 11.5 g, Fat: 9.3 g, Protein: 1.9 g, Fiber: 4.7 g.

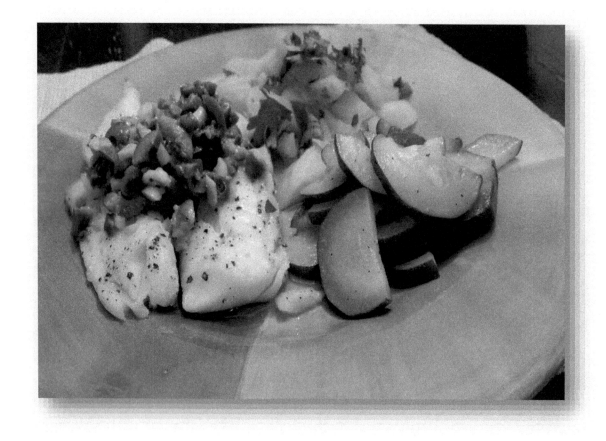

36. Easy Summer Vegetable Medley

Preparation time: 15 minutes

Cooking time: 6 hours

Servings: 6

Ingredients:

- 2 zucchinis, diced into 1-inch pieces
- 2 cups cauliflower florets
- 1 cup button mushrooms, halved
- 1 teaspoon dried thyme
- 1 yellow bell pepper, cut into strips
- ½ cup extra-virgin olive oil
- ¼ cup balsamic vinegar
- ¼ teaspoon salt

Directions:

1. Stir together the olive oil, vinegar, salt, and thyme in a large bowl until well combined.

2. Fold in the zucchini, cauliflower, mushrooms, and bell pepper strips, then toss until the vegetables are coated thoroughly.

3. Put the vegetables into the slow cooker and cook covered on LOW for about 6 hours, or until the vegetables are tender.

4. Let stand for 5 minutes and serve warm on a plate.

TIP: The balsamic vinegar can be replaced with the low-carb vinegars, such as apple cider vinegar or red wine vinegar.

Nutrition:

Calories: 186 | fat: 18.3g | protein: 1.2g

| net carbs: 4.1g |fiber: 1g | cholesterol: 0mg

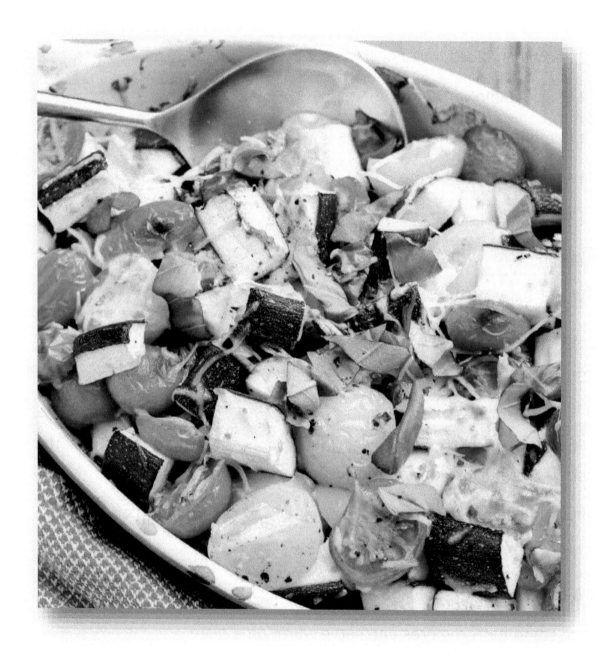

Chapter 8. Soups and Stews

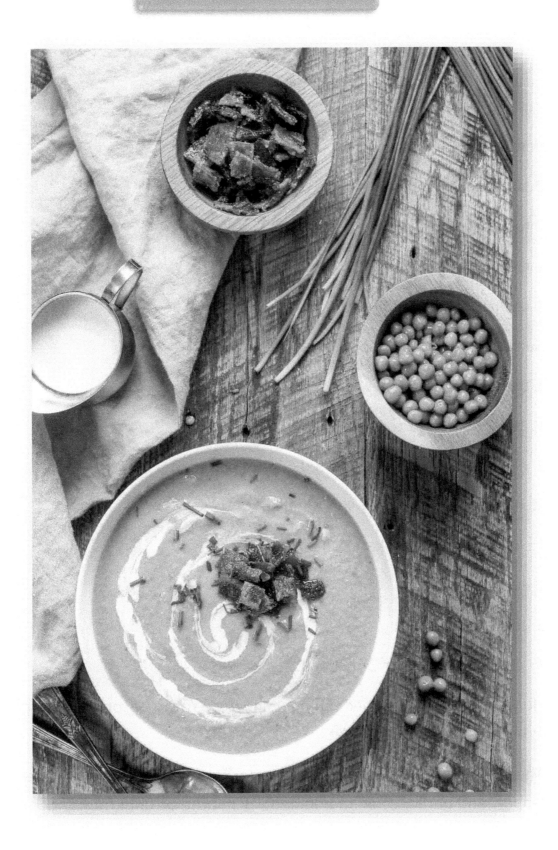

37. Bacon Green Soup

Preparation time: 15 minutes

Cooking time: 15 minutes

Servings: 4

Ingredients:

- 2 slices bacon, chopped
- 2 tablespoons scallions, chopped
- 1 carrot, chopped
- 1 celery, chopped
- Salt and ground black pepper, to taste
- 1 teaspoon garlic, finely chopped
- ½ teaspoon dried rosemary
- 1 sprig thyme, stripped and chopped
- ½ head green cabbage, shredded
- ½ head broccoli, broken into small florets
- 3 cups water
- 1 cup chicken stock
- ½ cup full-fat yogurt

Directions:

1. Heat a stockpot over medium heat; now, sear the bacon until crisp. Reserve the bacon and 1 tablespoon of fat.

2. Then, cook scallions, carrots, and celery in 1 tablespoon of reserved fat. Add salt, pepper, and garlic; cook an additional 1 minute or until fragrant.

3. Now, stir in rosemary, thyme, cabbage, and broccoli. Pour in water and stock, bringing to a rapid boil; reduce heat and let it simmer for 10 minutes more.

4. Add yogurt and cook an additional

5 minutes, stirring occasionally. Use an immersion blender, to purée your soup until smooth.

5. Taste and adjust the seasonings. Garnish with the cooked bacon just before serving.

Nutrition:

Calories: 96 fat: 7.7g protein: 3.0g carbs: 4.2g net carbs: 3.2g fiber: 1.0g

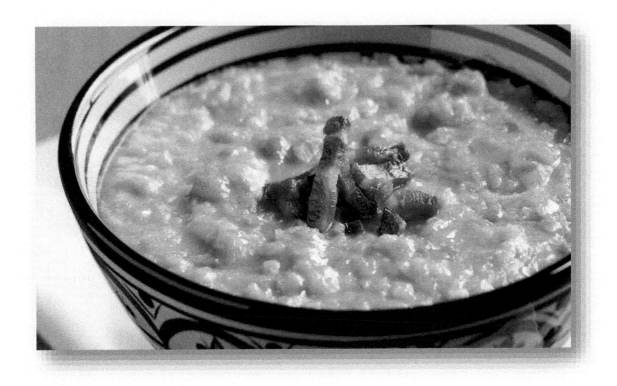

38. Zucchini and Celery Soup

Preparation time: 10 minutes

Cooking time: 15 minutes

Servings: 3

Ingredients:

- 2 teaspoons extra-virgin olive oil
- ½ pound (227 g) zucchini, peeled and diced
- ½ shallot, chopped
- ½ cup celery, chopped
- ½ teaspoon garlic powder
- ¼ teaspoon red pepper flakes
- 2 cups vegetable broth Directions:

1. Heat 1 teaspoon of the olive oil in a soup pot over medium-high heat; cook your zucchini for 1 to 2 minutes or until just tender; reserve.

2. In the same pot, heat the remaining teaspoon of olive oil; sauté the shallot until tender and translucent.

3. Add the remaining ingredients to the sautéed vegetables in the soup pot. Reduce the heat to medium-low, cover and let it cook for 15 minutes or until thoroughly heated.

4. Ladle into serving bowls and serve warm. Bon appétit!

Nutrition

Calories: 57 fat: 3.2g protein: 2.2g carbs: 3.6g net carbs: 2.5g fiber: 1.1g

39. Turkey Taco Soup

Preparation time: 10 minutes

Cooking time: 4 hours

Servings: 6

Ingredients:

- 1-pound (454 g) ground turkey
- 5 cups chicken bone broth (you can also use regular chicken broth)
- 1 cup canned diced tomatoes (no sugar added)
- 1 cup whipped cream cheese
- 1 yellow onion, chopped
- 1 tablespoon chili powder
- 1 teaspoon cumin
- 1 teaspoon garlic powder
- 1 teaspoon onion powder Directions:

1. Add all the ingredients to the base of a Crock-Pot minus the cream cheese and cover with the chicken broth.

2. Set on high and cook for 4 hours adding in the cream cheese at the 3.5- hour mark.

3. Stir well before serving. Nutrition:

Calories: 336 fat: 22.9g protein: 27.9g carbs: 5.9g net carbs: 4.8g fiber: 1.1g

40. Tomato Soup

Preparation time: 15 minutes

Cooking time: 10 minutes

Servings: 2

Ingredients:

- ½ of medium white onion, chopped
- 15 oz. canned diced tomatoes, with their juices
- 1 garlic clove, minced
- ¾ cup heavy cream
- 2 tablespoons basil leaves, julienned

Directions:

1. Put onion, tomatoes, garlic, and basil in a saucepan and stir well.

2. Cook over medium-high heat for about 10 minutes and transfer into an immersion blender.

3. Puree until smooth and mix in the heavy cream. Serve.

Nutrition:

Calories 207 Fat 17.1g

Cholesterol 62mg Sodium 29mg Carbs 12.7g Fiber 3.2g Sugars 6.8g Protein 3.3g

41. Cheesy Cauliflower Soup

Preparation time: 15 minutes

Cooking time: 16 minutes

Servings: 2

Ingredients:

- ½ of yellow onion
- 1 tablespoon butter
- 2 cups chicken broth
- 1/3 cup cheddar cheese, shredded
- 2 cups cauliflower, cut into florets

Directions:

1. Heat butter in a heavy pot and add onions. Sauté for about 3 minutes and add chicken broth and cauliflower.

2. Allow to simmer for about 10 minutes and transfer into an immersion blender. Blend until smooth and return to the pot.

3. Stir in the cheddar cheese and cook for about 3 minutes until the cheese is melted. Serve.

Nutrition:

Calories 201 Fat 13.5g

Cholesterol 35mg Sodium 952mg Carbs 9g

Fiber 3.1g Sugars 4.4g Protein 11.9g

42. Hot Mushroom Clear Soup

Preparation time: 15 minutes

Cooking time: 11 minutes

Servings: 2

Ingredients:

- 1 cup mushrooms, finely chopped
- 2 cups of water
- 1 tablespoon butter
- Salt, to taste
- Black pepper, to taste

Directions:

1. Heat butter in a heavy pot and add mushrooms. Cook on low heat for about 5 minutes and add water.

2. Season with salt and black pepper and cook for about 6 minutes, stirring occasionally. Scoop out into a bowl and serve hot.

Nutrition: Calories 59

Fat 5.9g Cholesterol 15mg Sodium 128mg Carbs 1.2g

Fiber 0.4g Sugars 0.6g Protein 1.2g

Chapter 9. Snacks

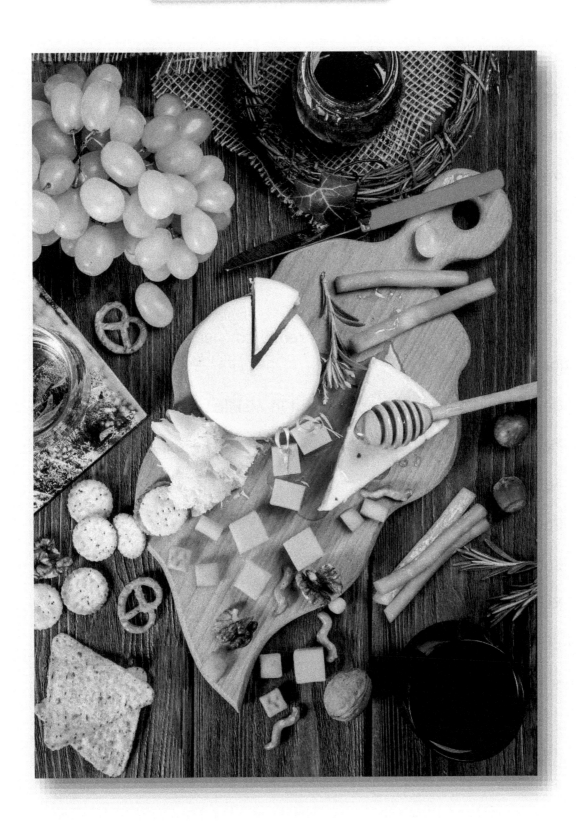

43. Country Style Chard

Preparation time: 2 minutes

Cooking Time: 3 minutes

Servings: 2

Ingredients:

- 4 slices bacon, chopped
- 2 tbsp butter
- 2 tbsp fresh lemon juice
- ½ tsp garlic paste
- 1 bunch Swiss chard, stems removed, leaves cut into 1-inch pieces

Directions:

1. On a medium heat, cook the bacon in a skillet until the fat begins to brown.
2. Melt the butter in the skillet and add the lemon juice and garlic paste.
3. Add the chard leaves and cook until they begin to wilt.
4. Cover and turn up the heat to high.
5. Cook for 3 minutes.
6. Mix well, sprinkle with salt and serve.

Nutrition:

Amount per one Servings: 190 cal., 4g fat, 5g protein & 10g carbs.

44. Bacon-Wrapped Sausage Skewers

Preparation time: 3 minutes

Cooking Time: 5 minutes

Servings: 2

Ingredients:

- 5 Italian chicken sausages
- 10 slices bacon Directions:

1. Preheat your deep fryer to 370°F/190°C.
2. Cut the sausage into four pieces.
3. Slice the bacon in half.
4. Wrap the bacon over the sausage.
5. Skewer the sausage.
6. Fry for 4-5 minutes until browned. Nutrition:

Amount per one Servings: 290 cal., 22g fat, 8g protein & 1g carbs.

45. Apple Crisp

Preparation Time: 5 minutes

Cooking Time: 2 minutes

Servings: 6

Ingredients:

- 5 cups sliced apples
- 1 1/2 cups vanilla chia granola
- 1/2 teaspoon ground ginger
- 1/2 lemon, zested
- 1/4 cup brown sugar
- 1 1/8 teaspoon cinnamon
- 2 tablespoons maple syrup
- 1 teaspoon vanilla extract, unsweetened
- 1/4 cup coconut oil
- 2/3 cup water
- Coconut whipped cream for serving Directions:

1. Take a small bowl, add granola into it along with 2 tablespoons sugar and coconut oil and stir until well combined.

2. Switch on the instant pot, place apples in the inner pot, sprinkle with remaining sugar, ginger, and 1 teaspoon cinnamon, drizzle with maple and vanilla, pour in water, spread the apple slices in an even layer and cover evenly with granola mixture.

3. Shut the pot with the lid in the sealed position, press the manual button, press the +/- button to set the cooking time to 2 minutes, press the pressure level to select the high-pressure setting, and let cook; the instant pot will take 10 minutes to preheat and then the timer will start.

4. When it's done and the timer beeps, release the pressure through quick pressure release; this will take 3 minutes, and then carefully move the vent to "venting."

5. Meanwhile, take a small bowl, add lemon zest and remaining cinnamon and stir until mixed.

6. Open the instant pot, let the apple crisp stand for 5 minutes until the sauce has thickened, and distribute it into bowls.

7. Garnish apple crisp with lemon zest mixture and serve with coconut whipped cream.

Nutrition: Calories 293, Fat 13, Carbs 13,

Protein 4

46. Sugar Snap Bacon

Preparation time: 7 minutes

Cooking Time: 3 minutes

Servings: 4

Ingredients:

- 3 cups sugar snap peas
- ½ tbsp lemon juice
- 2 tbsp bacon fat
- 2 tsp garlic
- ½ tsp red pepper flakes

Directions:

1. In a skillet, cook the bacon fat until it begins to smoke.
2. Add the garlic and cook for 2 minutes.
3. Add the sugar peas and lemon juice.
4. Cook for 2-3 minutes.
5. Remove and sprinkle with red pepper flakes and lemon zest.
6. Serve!

Nutrition:

Amount per one Servings: 80 cal., 4g fat, 3g protein & 1g carbs.

Chapter 10. Desserts

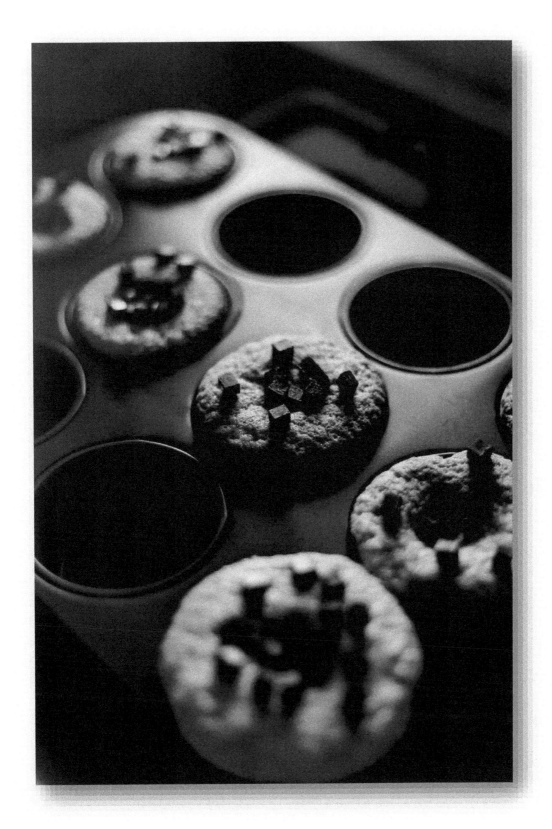

47. Chocolate Peanut Butter Ice Cream Bars

Preparation Time: 4 hours and 20 minutes

Cooking time: 0 minutes

Servings: 15 Ingredients

- 1 cup heavy whipping cream
- 1 tsp vanilla extract
- ¾ tsp xanthan gum
- 1/3 cup peanut butter
- 1 cup half and half
- 1 ½ cups almond milk
- 1/3 tsp stevia powder
- 1 tbsp vegetable glycerin
- 3 tbsp xylitol

Chocolate:

- ¾ cup coconut oil
- ¼ cup cocoa butter pieces, chopped
- 2 ounces chocolate, unsweetened
- 3 ½ tsp super sweet blend Directions:

1. Blend all of the ice cream ingredients until smooth.
2. Place in an ice cream maker and follow the instructions.
3. Spread the ice cream into a lined pan, and freeze for about 4 hours.

4. Combine all of the chocolate ingredients in a microwave-safe bowl and microwave until melted. Slice the ice cream bars.

5. Dip them into the cooled chocolate mixture.

Nutrition:

Per Serving Calories 345 Net Carbs 5g, Fat 32g, Protein 4g

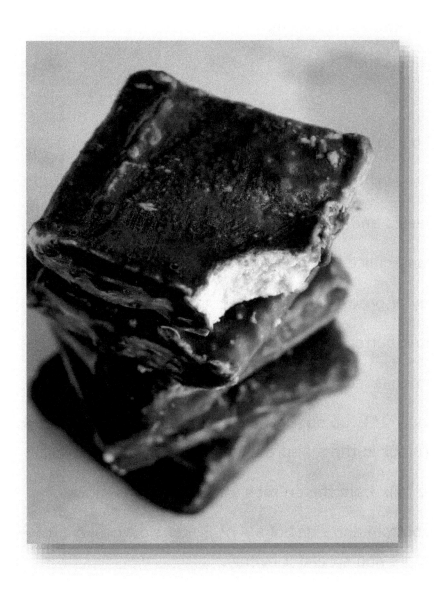

48. Crockpot Apple Pudding Cake

Preparation time: 20 min

Cooking time: 3 hours

Servings: 10

Ingredients

- 2 cups all-purpose flour
- 2/3 cup plus ¼ cup divided sugar
- 3 tsp of baking soda
- 1 tsp salt
- ½ cup cold butter
- 1 cup milk
- 4 apples, peeled and diced
- 1 ½ cup orange juice
- ½ cup honey or brown sugar
- 2 Tbsp melted butter
- 1 tsp cinnamon Directions:

1. Combine flour, 2/3 cup sugar, baking powder, and salt. Cut the butter until you have thick crumbs in the mixture.

2. Remove the milk from the crumbs until it becomes moist.

3. Grease the bottom and sides of a 4 or 5-liter slow cooker. Place the dough at the bottom of the pot and spread it evenly.

4. Beat the orange juice, honey, butter, remaining sugar and cinnamon in a medium pan. Decorate the apples.

5. Place the jar opening with a clean cloth, place the lid. Prevents condensation on the cover from reaching the pot. Place the pan on top and cook until apples are tender for 2 to 3 hours.

Nutrition: Cal 405 Fat 9 g Saturated fat 3 g Carbs 79 g Fiber 2 g Sugar 63 g Protein 3 g

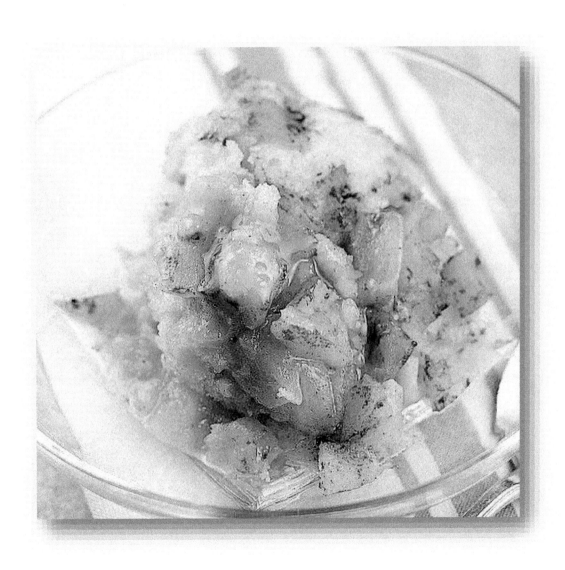

49. Mocha Ice Bombs

Preparation time: 2 hours

Cooking time: 10 minutes

Servings: 4

Ingredients

- ½ pound cream cheese
- 4 tbsp d sweetener, powdered
- 2 ounces strong coffee
- 2 tbsp cocoa powder, unsweetened
- 1-ounce cocoa butter, melted
- 2 ½ ounces dark chocolate, melted

Directions:

1. Combine cream cheese, sweetener, coffee, and cocoa powder in a food processor.

2. Roll 2 tbsp of the mixture and place on a lined tray.

3. Mix the cocoa butter and chocolate, and coat the bombs with it. Freeze for 2 hours.

Nutrition: Per Serving Calories 127, Net Carbs 1.4g, Fat 13g, Protein 1.9g

50. Dark Chocolate Almond Bark

Preparation time: 1 hour Cooking time: 15 minutes Servings: 12

Ingredients

- ½ cup almonds
- ½ cup coconut butter
- 10 drops stevia
- ¼ tsp salt
- ½ cup coconut flakes, unsweetened
- 4 ounces dark chocolate Directions:

1. Preheat the oven to 350 F.
2. Place the almonds in a baking sheet, and toast for 5 minutes.
3. Melt together the butter and chocolate. Stir in stevia.
4. Line a cookie sheet with waxed paper and spread the chocolate evenly.
5. Scatter the almonds on top and sprinkle with salt.
6. Refrigerated for one hour. Nutrition

Per Serving Calories 161, Net Carbs 2g, Fat 15.3g, Protein 2g

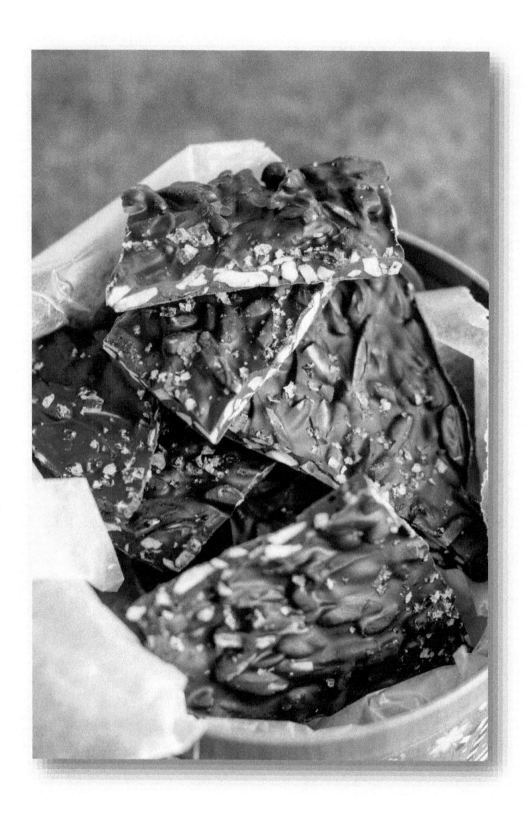

Conclusion

Thank you for making it to the end. The Keto Diet Recipes is a series of balanced recipes for those involved in a ketogenic diet. A team of health experts has carefully designed each recipe to ensure that it is as nutritious as possible.

The KETO DIET RECIPES is an excellent guide for those on a low-carb or ketogenic diet. If you're new to the diet or just want a fast keto meal option that doesn't require much effort, the KETO DIET RECIPES is a must-have. This cookbook will illustrate how easy it is to prepare delectable meals using just a few simple ingredients.

The ketogenic diet emphasizes the intake of whole foods while avoiding processed foods. Many people find it difficult to sustain a low-carb diet without getting hungry, but there are plenty of paleo recipes that can help. By integrating prepared sauces, soups, and stews into your meals, you can fulfill your cravings in a number of ways. Using frozen foods saves time in the kitchen and lets you keep on board with your meal plan when you feel like you're going off track.

The Keto Diet is a low-carbohydrate, high-fat diet. This diet, however, may not be for you if you have problems with your metabolism or have metabolic disorders such as diabetes. Since this is not a strict carb-free diet, it is important to talk with your doctor before beginning. Obesity and insulin resistance, as well as epilepsy and mitochondrial disorders like type 1 and type 2 diabetes, are the best candidates for the ketogenic diet. This diet has several different variants, but this one focuses on reducing carbohydrates that the body cannot use or metabolize for energy (glycogen). This decreases blood glucose levels to dangerously low levels and improves fat metabolism, allowing us to turn to our fat reserves for energy instead of carbs. As a result, it facilitates weight loss from fat reserves rather than muscle mass, making the body leaner and more defined when encouraging weight loss rather than gain, which can be more risky when attempting to lose weight. The concept behind keto is that the body would burn its own fat reserves for energy rather than depleting useful carbohydrate stores first.

They all follow such standards, such as the Keto Diet's specifications as well as other essential criteria including being low in carbs and high in fat. The recipes contain a wide variety of ingredients, allowing you to mix and match according to your personal preferences. The range of recipes included in this Keto Diet Recipes will astound you.

This isn't just a cookbook, though. The KETO DIET RECIPES is a series of helpful suggestions and information to help you stick to your diet plan. That is why we built it. We want you to be happy in your keto journey so you can lose weight and meet your health goals!

The ketogenic diet has piqued the interest of many people. This diet was designed to help children with epilepsy manage their seizures, but it has since gained widespread popularity.

The ketogenic diet limits carbohydrate consumption and forces your body to burn fat for energy. A low-carbohydrate diet has been shown in research to help people lose weight and regulate their blood sugar levels.

I hope you have learned something!!!

Note:

CPSIA information can be obtained
at www.ICGtesting.com
Printed in the USA
BVHW051324150421
605032BV00002B/289